Fighting Deadly Diseases

Carmel Reilly

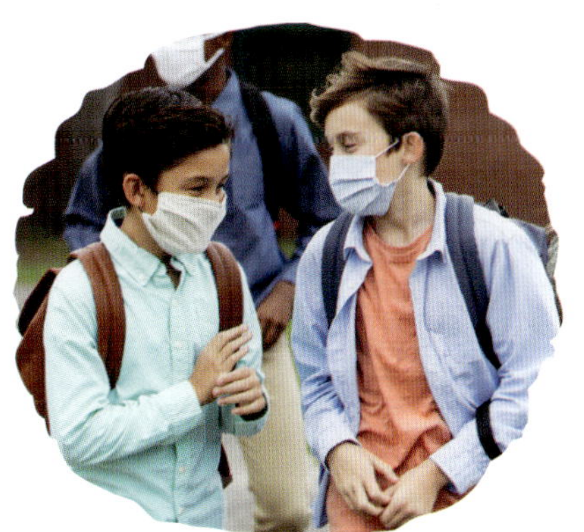

Contents

Fighting Deadly Diseases

Dangerous Diseases

There is nothing that can affect human life more than disease. Some diseases, such as cancer, target one person at a time and cannot be spread to others. However, there are many diseases that can be passed on either from person to person, or from insects and animals.

Diseases that can be caught from others are called "infectious" diseases. Although many infectious diseases can be mild, such as colds, others, such as malaria, can be deadly. For most of human history, infectious diseases have been the most dangerous illnesses.

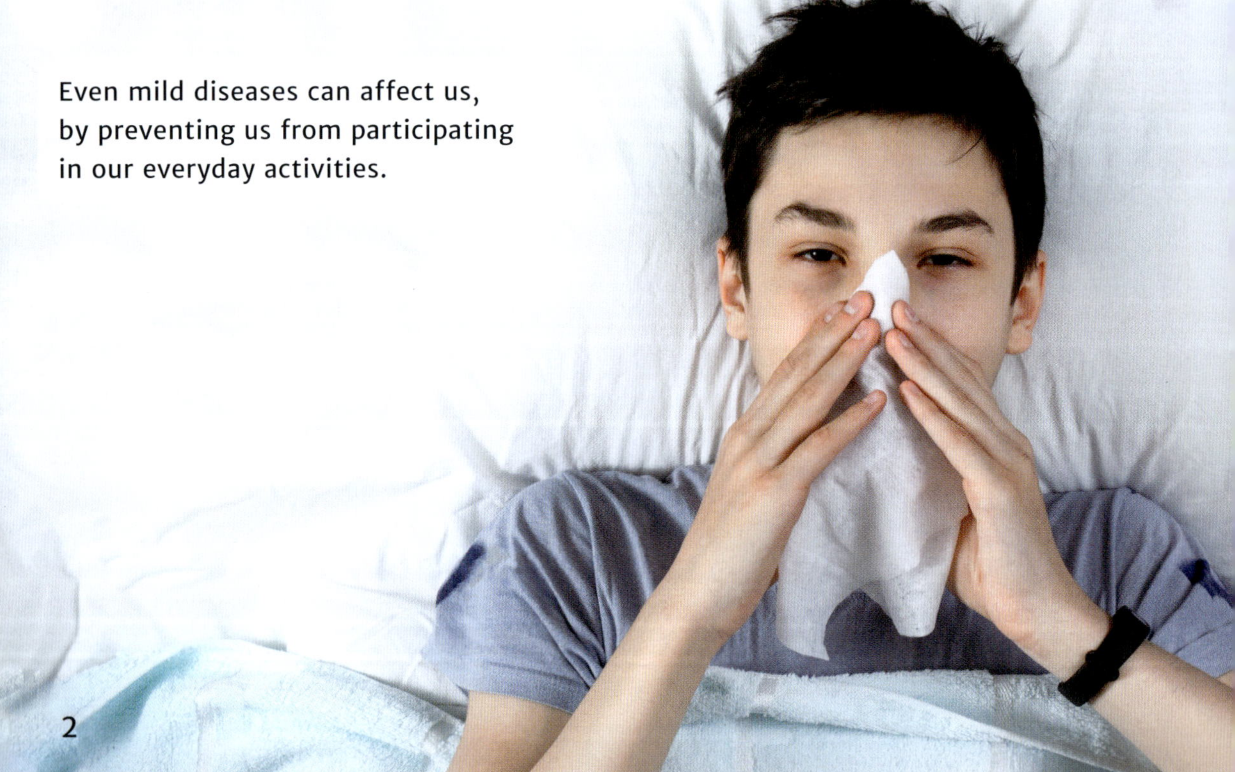

Even mild diseases can affect us, by preventing us from participating in our everyday activities.

Infectious diseases are caused by germs, which are tiny life forms that can only be seen with a microscope, such as **bacteria**, **viruses** and **parasites**. Once germs enter the human body, they can begin to damage certain parts of it. This damage leads to people having **symptoms** of an illness. Symptoms often include fevers, coughing, rashes, aches and pains, headaches and vomiting.

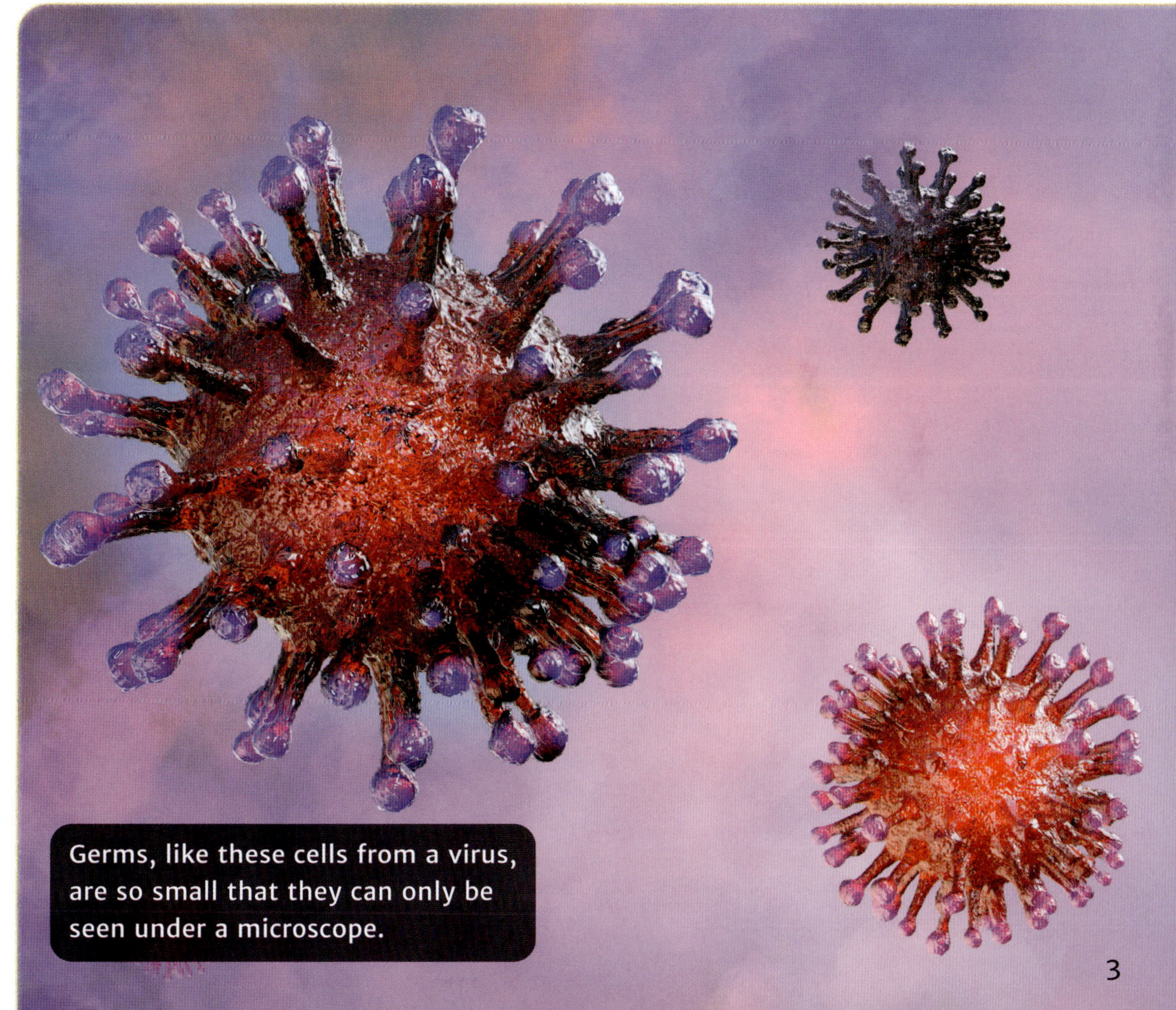

Germs, like these cells from a virus, are so small that they can only be seen under a microscope.

Before the 1900s

Until the twentieth century, infectious diseases killed more people than any other cause of death. Before the 1900s, most people had poor diets, worked unsafe jobs and lived in overcrowded housing. Water supplies were often unclean, and only a few places had **sewerage** systems to clear waste. Unhealthy environments meant infectious diseases could spread easily. In addition, people did not know about the importance of **hygiene** for killing germs, and there were no drug treatments or **vaccines**. The only way to stop a disease from spreading was to keep sick people apart from others, or for many people to become immune after recovering from a disease.

The immune system is a network, made up of cells in different parts of the body, that works to protect the body from bacteria and viruses that can cause illness. When a person recovers from a disease or receives a vaccine, they can become immune to it. Having immunity to a disease means they will not get the disease again, or will only get it mildly.

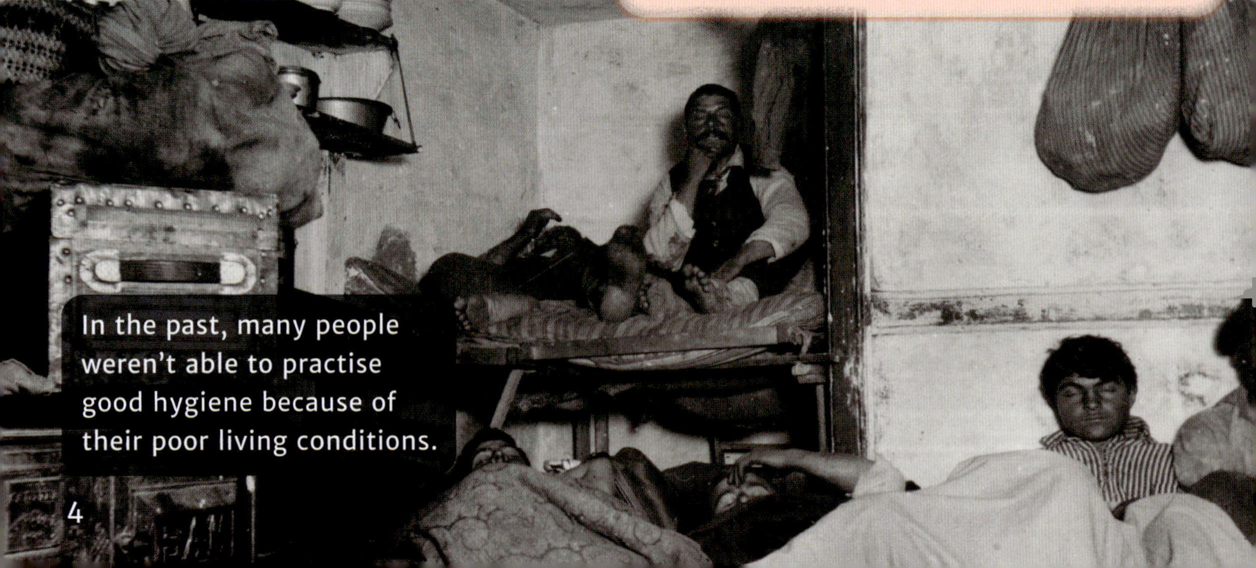

In the past, many people weren't able to practise good hygiene because of their poor living conditions.

Infectious Diseases Today

Over the past two centuries, hygiene has improved and people have generally become healthier. Scientific breakthroughs have also helped people to understand more about infectious diseases and how to stop their spread. As a result, bubonic plague is now rarely seen, and smallpox has been wiped out. However, other diseases, such as tuberculosis (TB), are still affecting millions of people every year, and new diseases, such as Covid-19, will keep appearing.

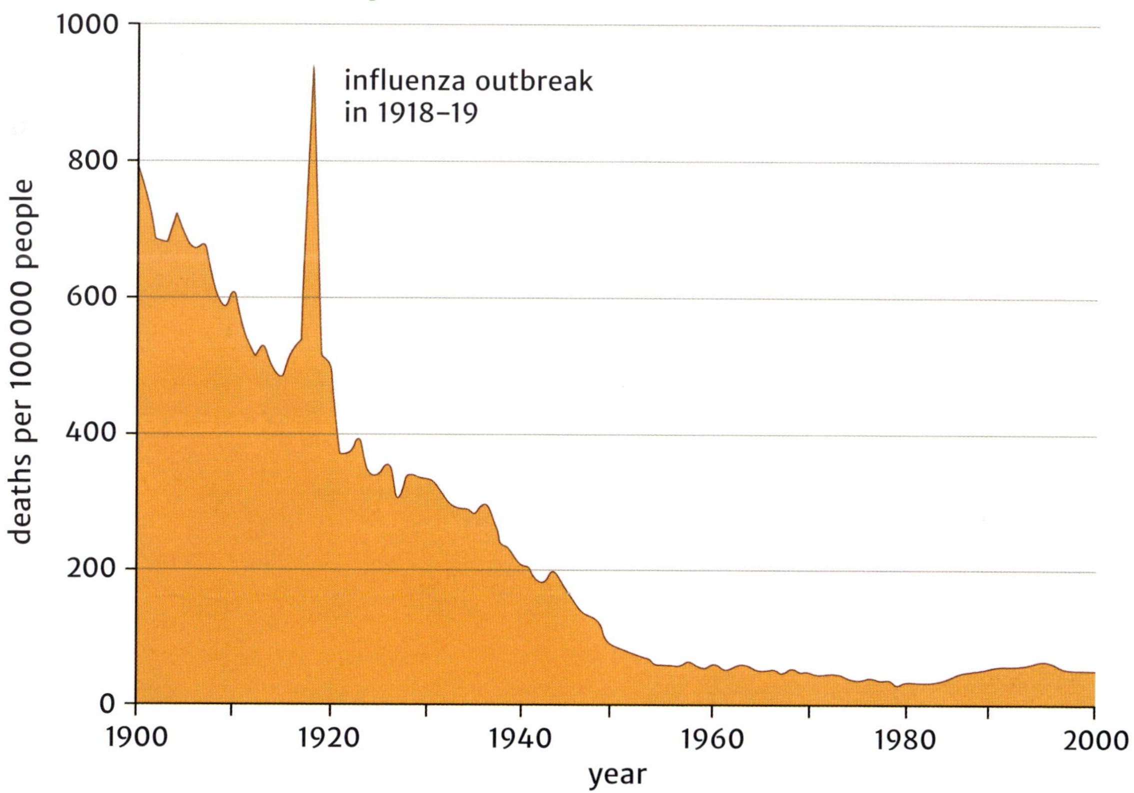

Major Deadly Diseases

For most of human history, infectious diseases from bubonic plague to influenza have caused millions of deaths. But in the past hundred years or so, people have found several ways to fight back.

Bubonic Plague

Bubonic plague is a deadly infectious disease that has taken the lives of hundreds of millions of people over thousands of years. People can catch bubonic plague through contact with infected, or diseased, animals, or from being bitten by parasites such as fleas that have fed on infected animals. Symptoms of bubonic plague include high fever, cramps, and swelling and pain in certain parts of the body.

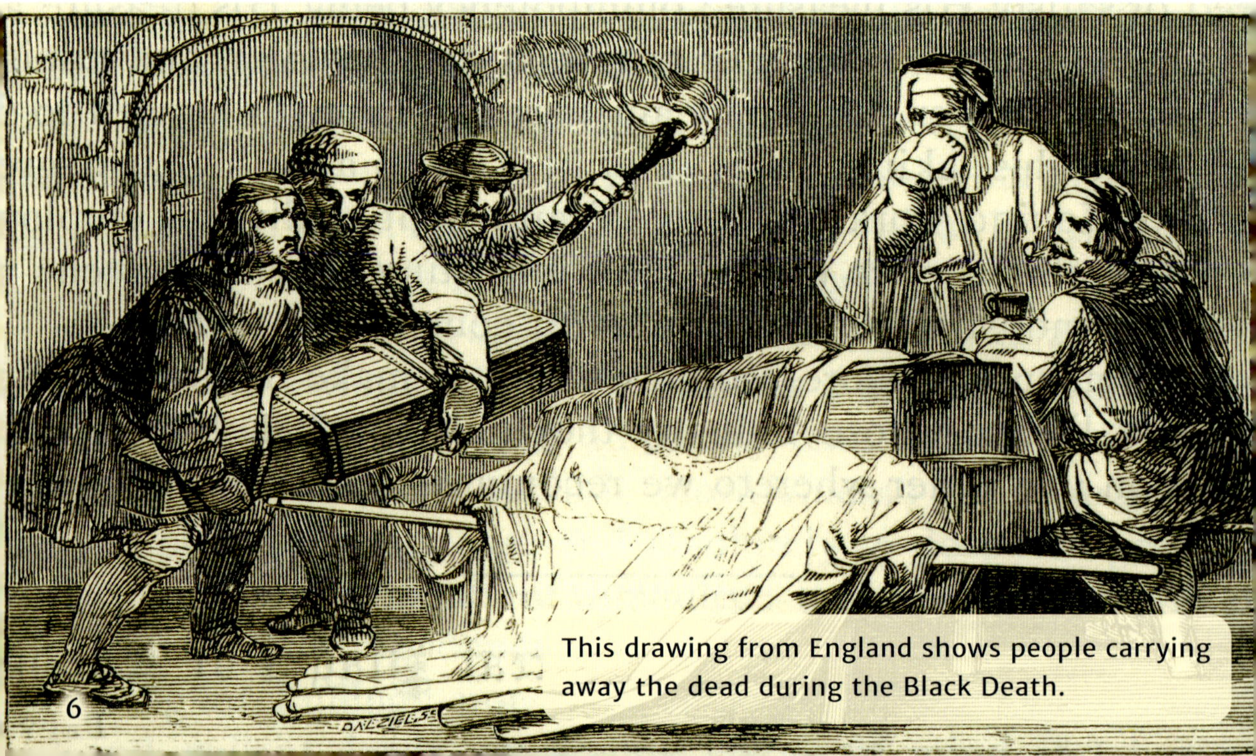

This drawing from England shows people carrying away the dead during the Black Death.

Bubonic Plague over Time

Scientists believe that bubonic plague has existed for around 5000 years. It was first written about in the 500s **CE** following a large outbreak, or **pandemic**, that affected the Mediterranean, a region covering southern Europe and northern Africa. This pandemic lasted for around 200 years and might have killed 25 million to 100 million people.

The largest known outbreak, also known as the "Black Death", occurred in the 1300s in the Middle East and Europe. It is believed to have wiped out a third of Europe's population. The last major outbreak started in Hong Kong and spread to various seaports around the world between 1894 and 1922.

It is believed that the name "Black Death" referred to the blackening of the skin in some people who caught bubonic plague.

During the Black Death, doctors would wear special masks that they thought would protect them from catching the disease.

Alexandre Yersin's Discovery

In 1894, Swiss-born French scientist Alexandre Yersin identified the type of bacteria that causes bubonic plague in humans and rats. His research led to the discovery that bubonic plague can be passed on to humans by the fleas that live on rats. Once people understood how bubonic plague spread, they were able to control it by cleaning up rubbish and reducing the numbers of rats and parasites. Improvements in hygiene, such as handwashing, also stopped the spread of bacterial germs.

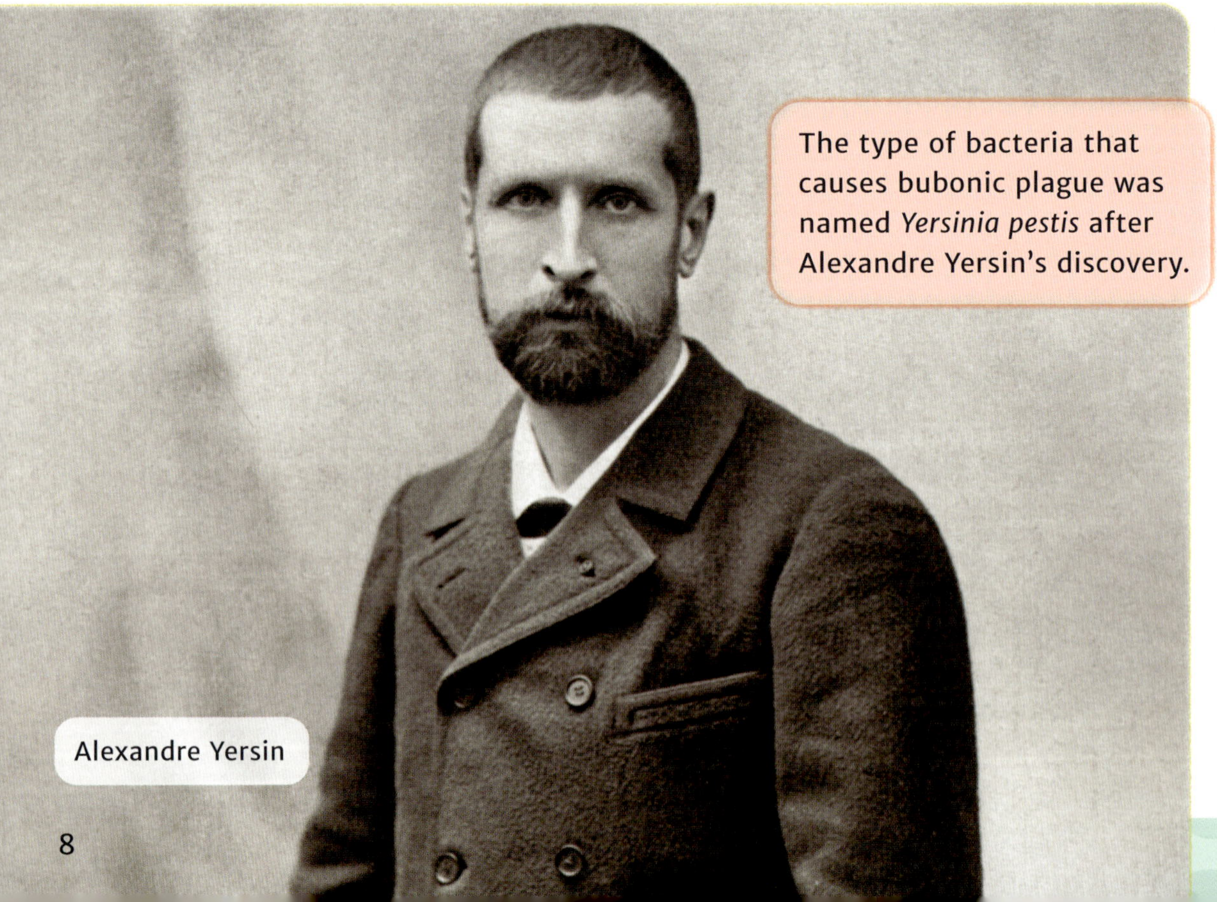

The type of bacteria that causes bubonic plague was named *Yersinia pestis* after Alexandre Yersin's discovery.

Alexandre Yersin

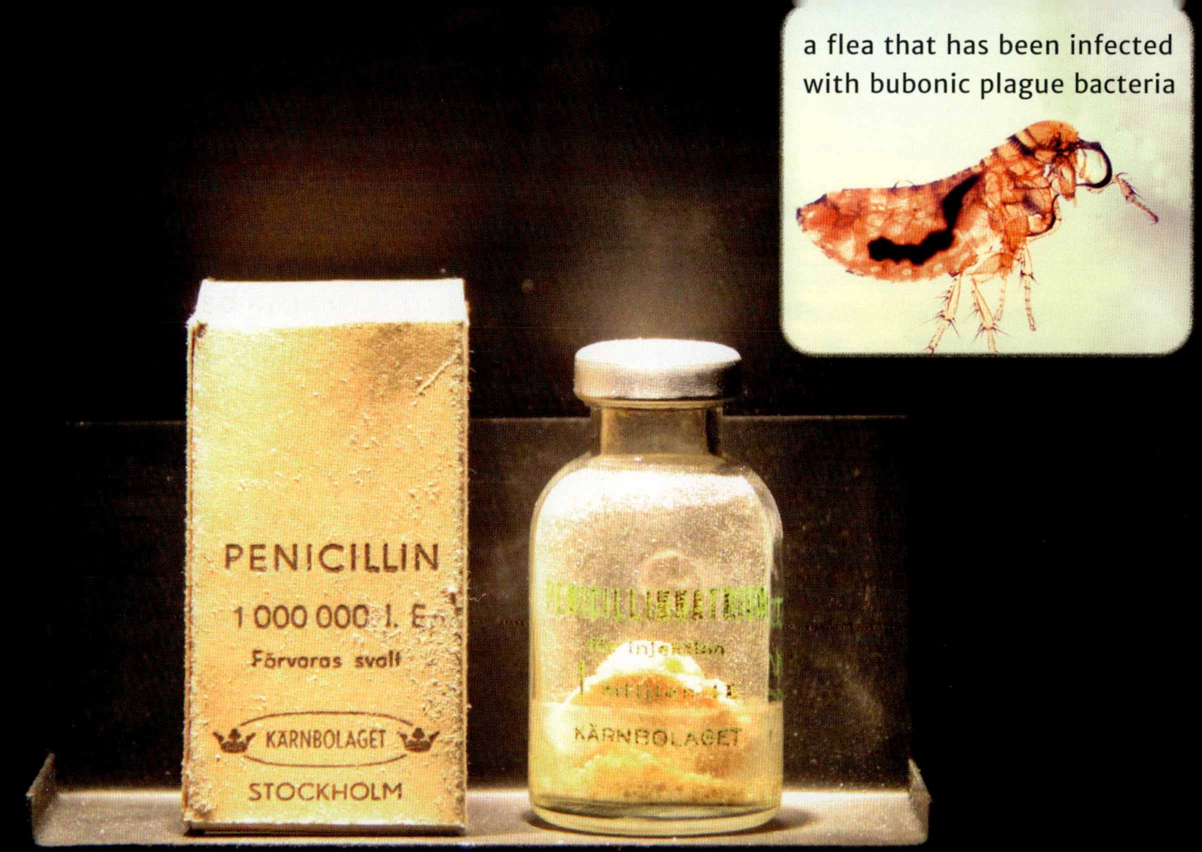

a flea that has been infected with bubonic plague bacteria

one of the first bottles of penicillin, a type of antibiotic

Bubonic Plague Today

Today, due to better public health and hygiene, outbreaks of bubonic plague are rare in most countries. The outbreaks that do occur are usually in rural areas, where it is easier for people to be bitten by infected animals. Since the 1940s, people who catch bubonic plague can be successfully treated with **antibiotics**, which are drugs that kill bacteria. This means that it is rarely deadly.

Smallpox

For many centuries, smallpox was one of the world's deadliest diseases. Around one in every three people who caught the illness did not survive. Smallpox was caused by a virus, a type of germ. The smallpox virus was passed from one person to another through the air, by people coughing and breathing. When people first became infected, they could have a fever, tiredness, and aches and pains. After a few days, these symptoms passed and were followed by a rash, which turned into large, pus-filled blisters that covered the head and body. These blisters often left survivors with badly scarred skin, and they could sometimes cause blindness.

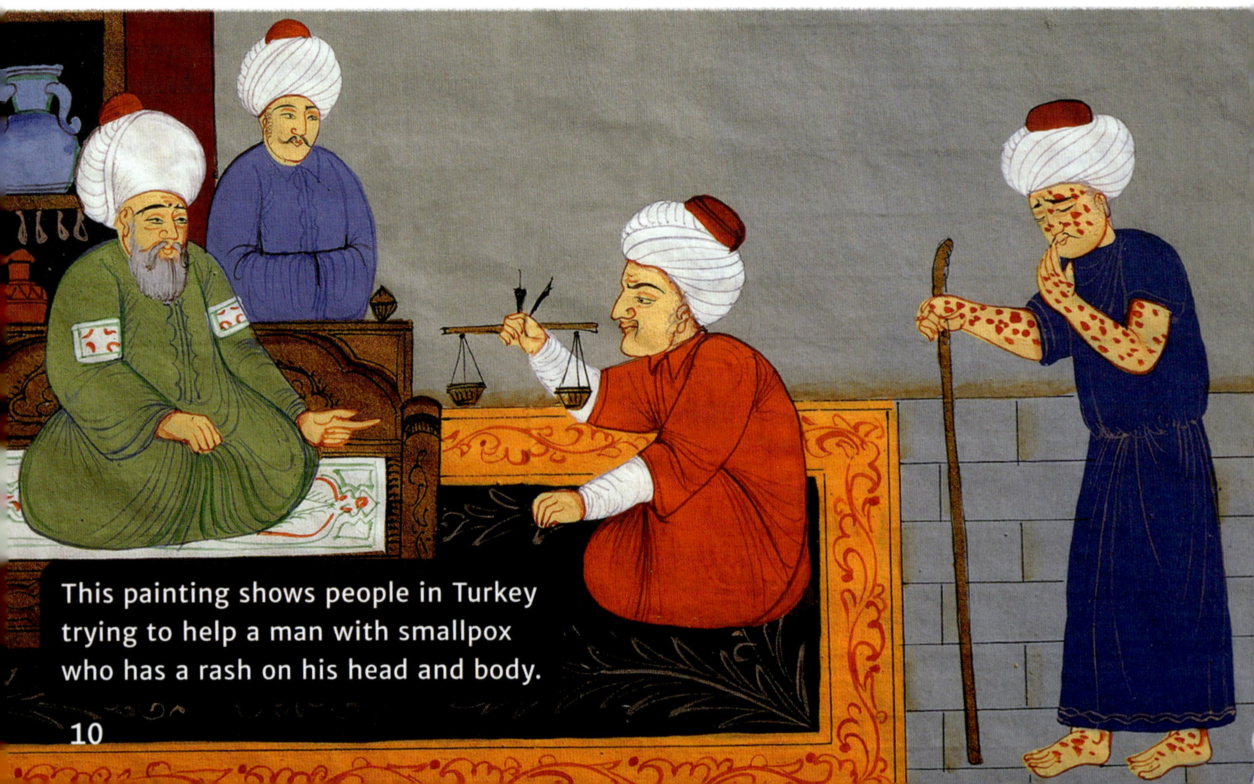

This painting shows people in Turkey trying to help a man with smallpox who has a rash on his head and body.

Smallpox over Time

Over a period of about 3000 years, waves of smallpox swept across Asia, the Middle East, Europe, the Americas and Africa, wiping out millions of people. In the 1700s, it is believed there were about 400 000 smallpox deaths in Europe every year. Even in the twentieth century, around 300 million people around the world died from the illness.

QUARANTINE
KEEP OUT
SMALL POX
Exists in these Premises
This Sign MUST NOT BE REMOVED
Without Permission of Health Officer
Date
M. D.
Health Officer

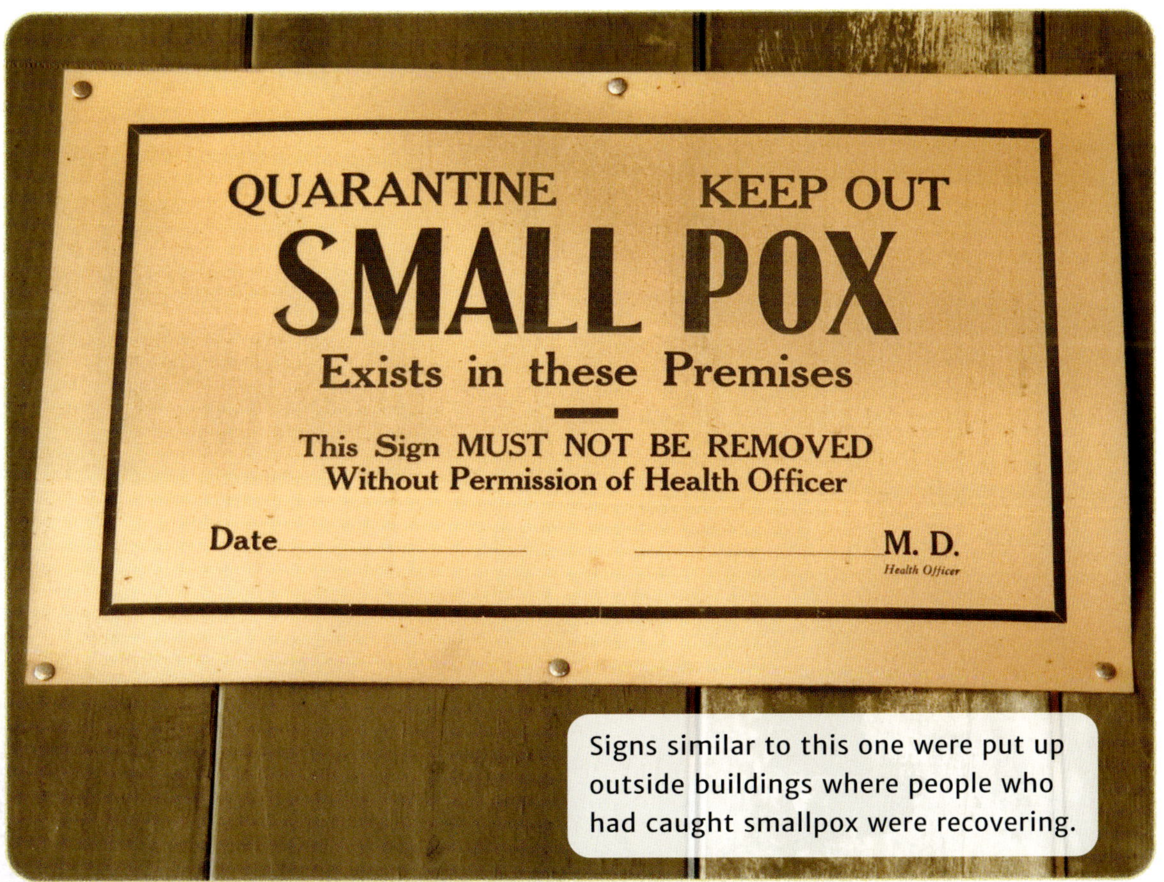

Signs similar to this one were put up outside buildings where people who had caught smallpox were recovering.

Edward Jenner's Vaccine Breakthrough

Edward Jenner was an English country doctor practising in the late 1700s. He noticed that patients who worked with animals often caught a mild disease called "cowpox". Recovering from cowpox seemed to give these patients immunity against smallpox. Edward Jenner experimented by injecting a patient with small amounts of cowpox and found that it protected them from getting smallpox. He called this process "vaccination".

Vaccination is a treatment that can give a person immunity to a disease. The word "vaccination" comes from the Latin word *vacca*, meaning cow.

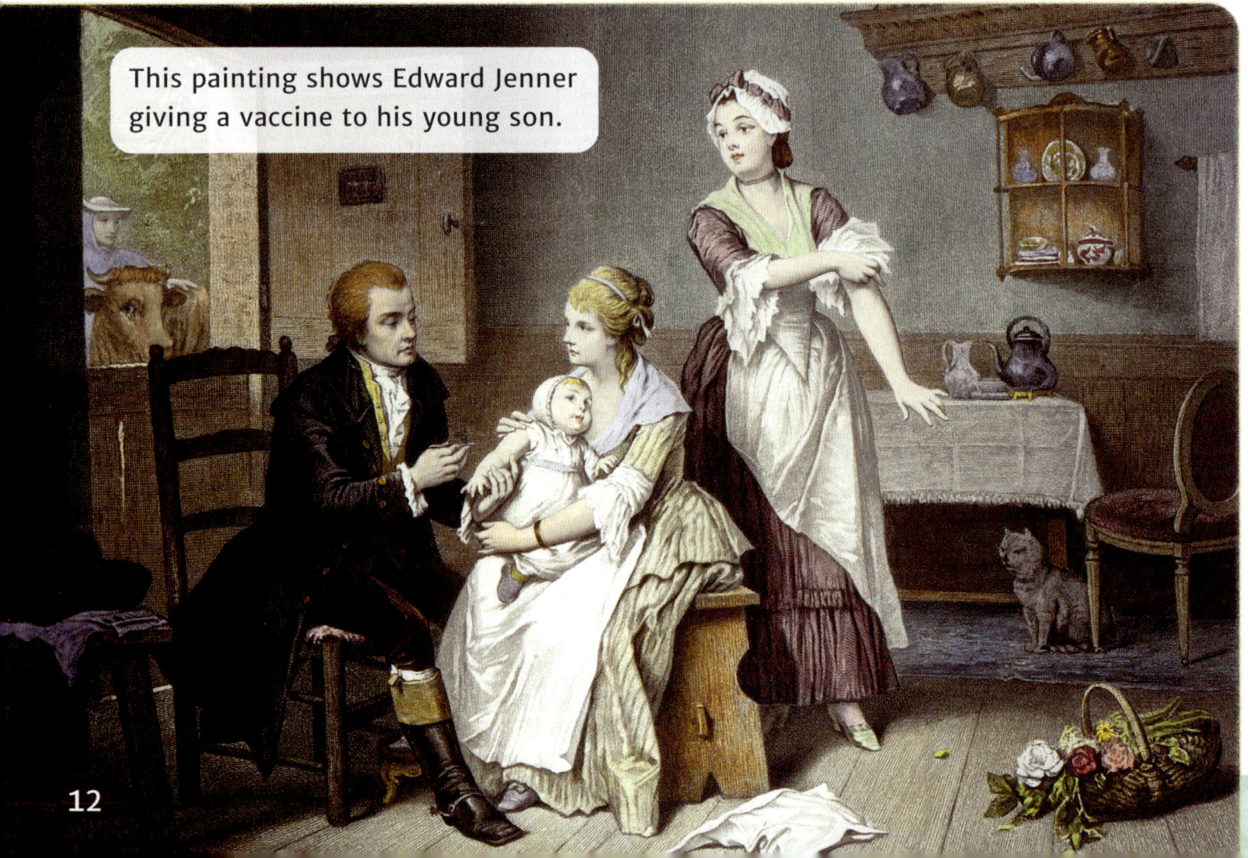

This painting shows Edward Jenner giving a vaccine to his young son.

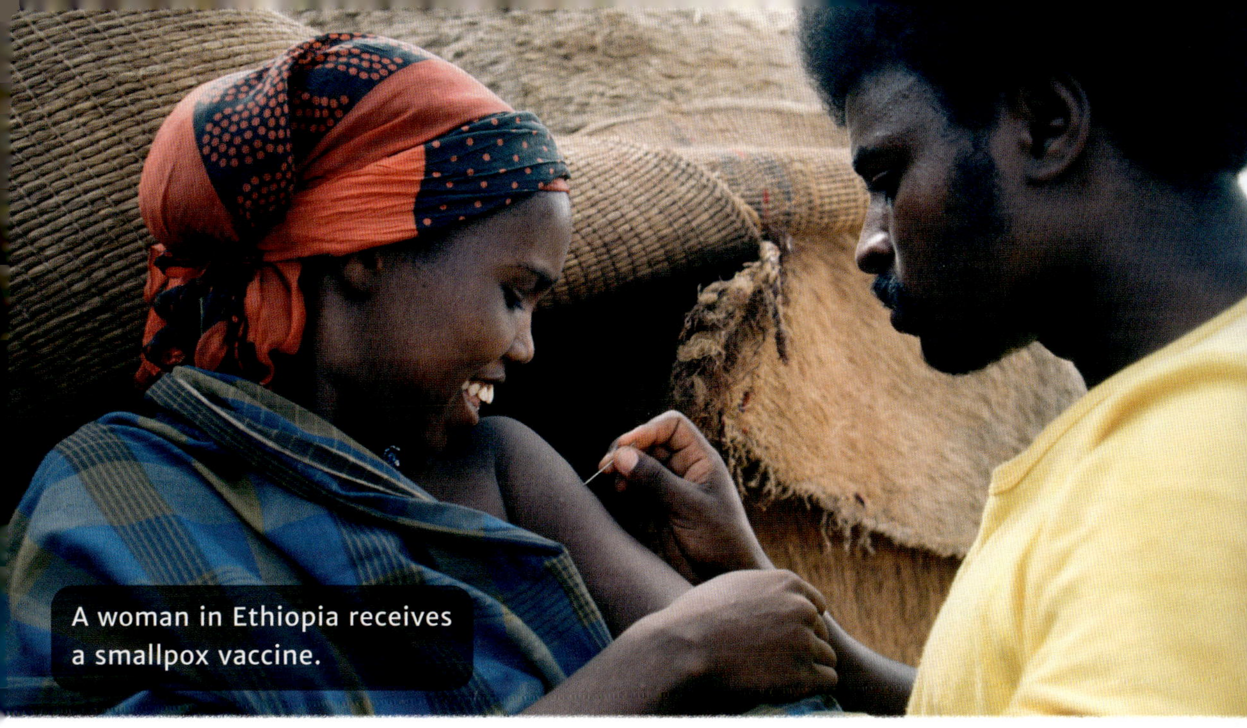

A woman in Ethiopia receives a smallpox vaccine.

The End of Smallpox

Over the next hundred years, the practice of vaccination spread. In most parts of the world, the numbers of people getting smallpox began to drop. However, the disease still remained a problem in some countries. In the mid-twentieth century, the **World Health Organization (WHO)** fought to end smallpox by vaccinating as many people as possible. In 1980, smallpox became the first deadly disease to be defeated by modern medicine.

The World Health Organization (WHO) is an international health agency that aims to create the best possible public health worldwide. Its work includes research, developing disease treatments and helping countries with their health programs.

Tuberculosis

Tuberculosis, or TB, is one of the world's most deadly infectious diseases. TB is caused by bacteria that spread through the air from person to person by talking, sneezing and coughing. Although large numbers of people catch TB, most of them live with the disease and never have symptoms. However, about one in ten infected people can become sick and infect others. The symptoms of TB include coughing, fever, tiredness and weight loss. Unlike some infectious diseases, TB does not appear in quick, deadly waves. Instead, it spreads slowly from person to person.

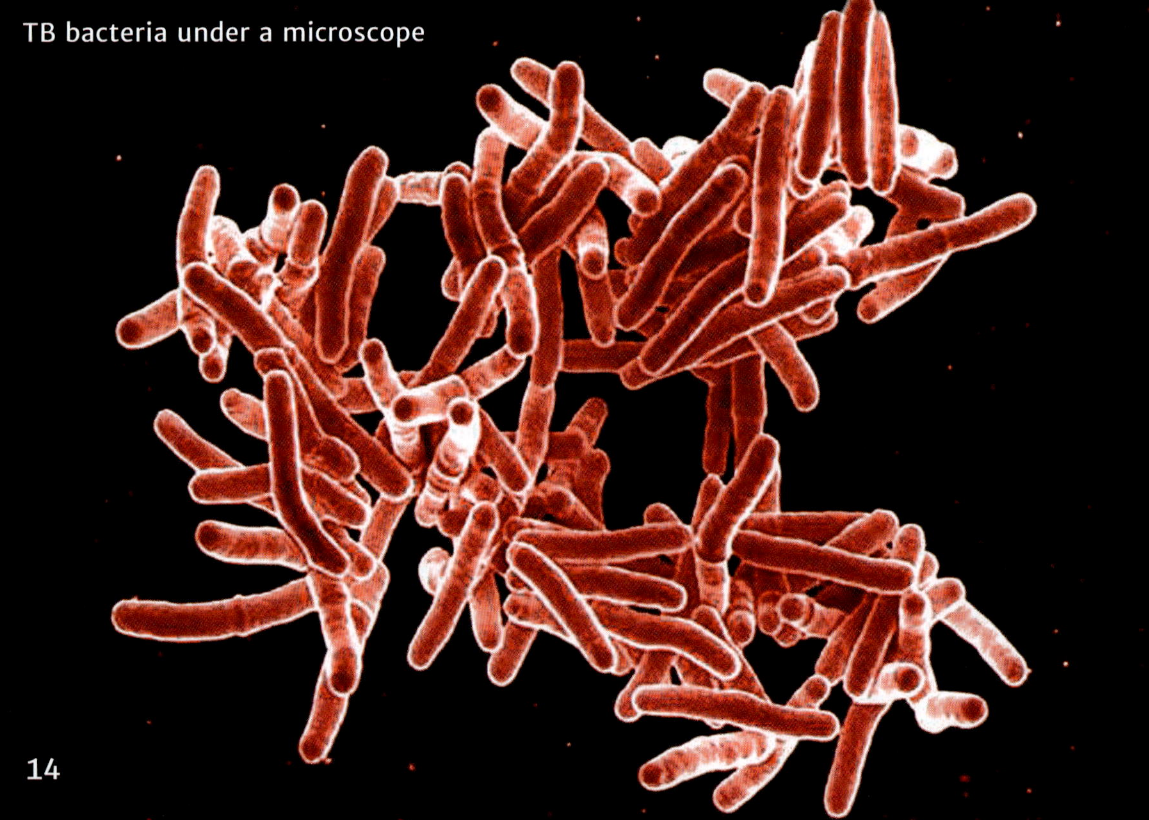
TB bacteria under a microscope

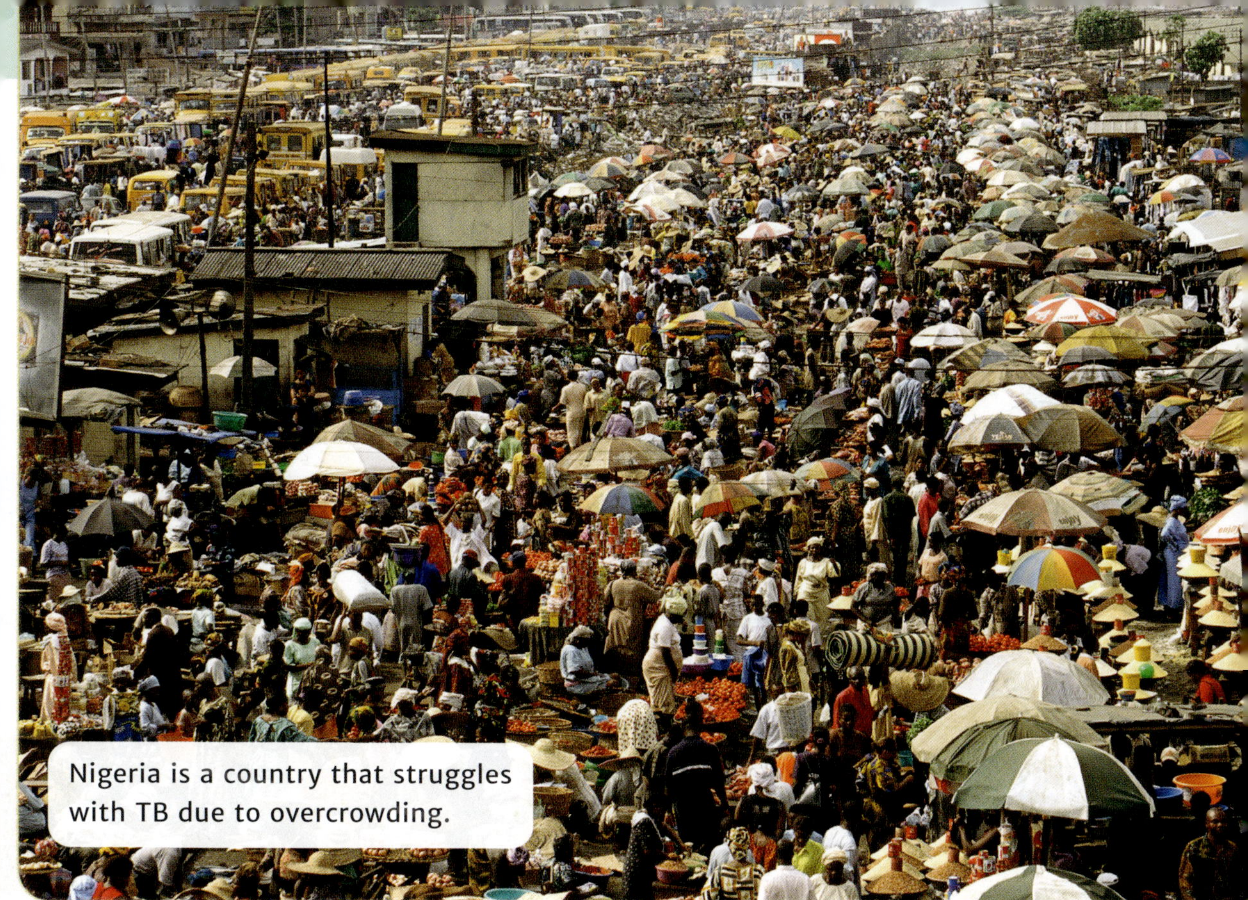

Nigeria is a country that struggles with TB due to overcrowding.

Tuberculosis over Time

TB has existed for thousands of years, but it became more widespread as towns and cities became larger, forcing people to live closer together. Between the 1600s and 1800s, TB caused 25 per cent of all deaths in Europe. TB is now rare in places such as Australia, the USA and Europe. However, it is still common in some parts of the world where housing is overcrowded and the healthcare system is weak. Worldwide, there are close to two billion people who have TB, and 4000 people die from this disease every day.

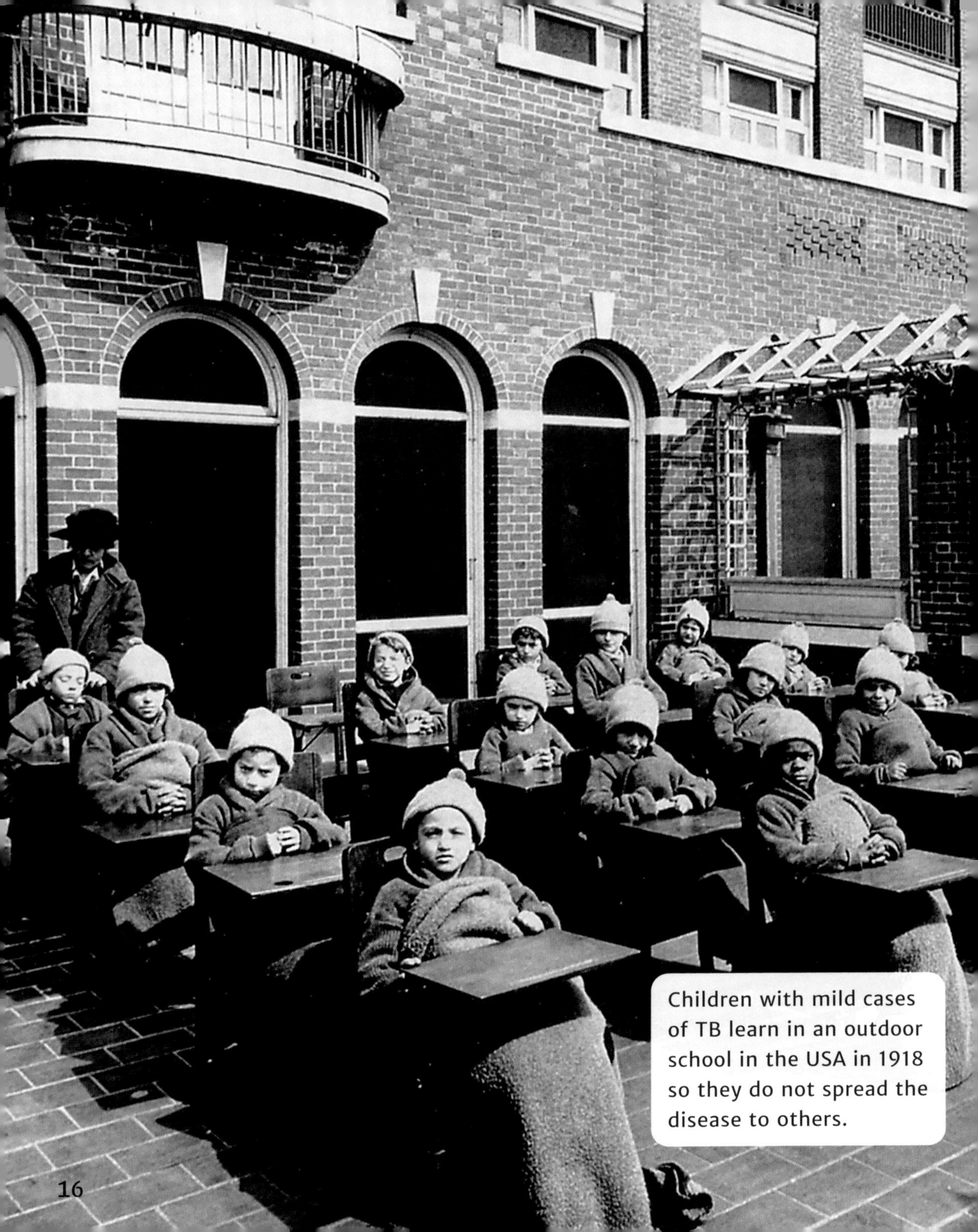

Children with mild cases of TB learn in an outdoor school in the USA in 1918 so they do not spread the disease to others.

Treatments for Tuberculosis

Since the late 1800s, the number of people that catch TB every year has fallen. This change has mainly been due to better food and hygiene, and housing that is less crowded. In the 1940s, antibiotics, or antibacterial drugs, began to be produced. They became the first successful treatment against TB, although they do not always work against the bacteria.

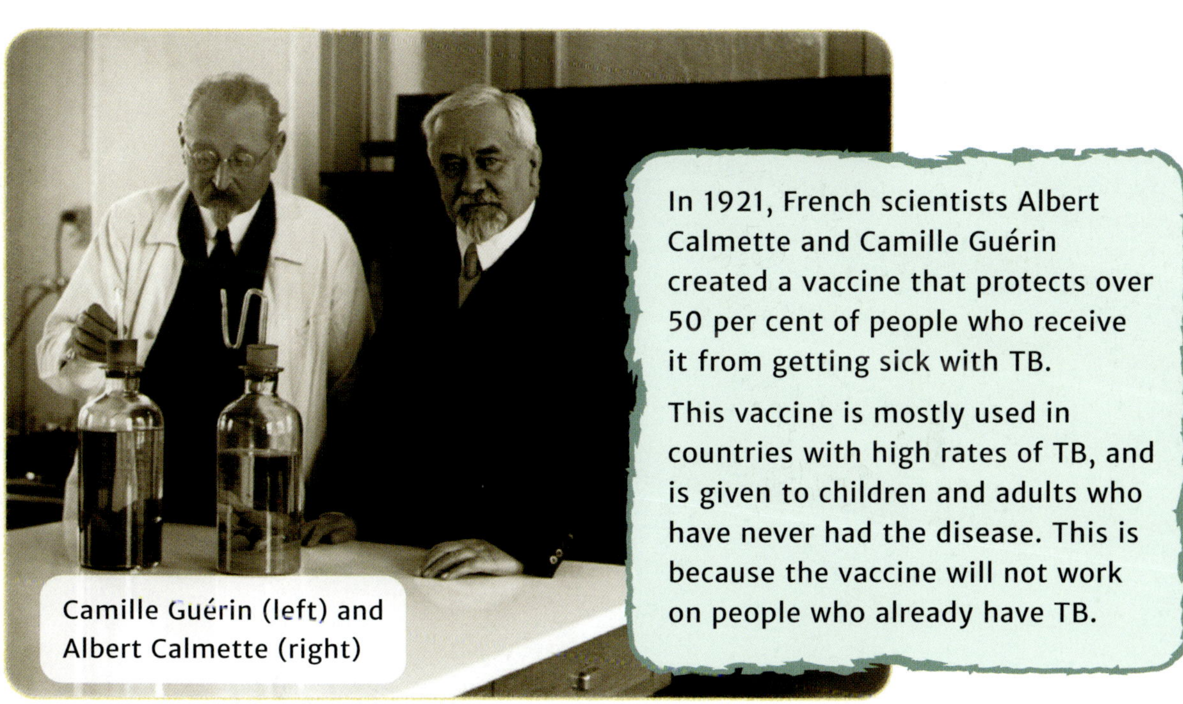

Camille Guérin (left) and Albert Calmette (right)

In 1921, French scientists Albert Calmette and Camille Guérin created a vaccine that protects over 50 per cent of people who receive it from getting sick with TB.

This vaccine is mostly used in countries with high rates of TB, and is given to children and adults who have never had the disease. This is because the vaccine will not work on people who already have TB.

While TB remains a major disease in about 30 countries around the world, the number of people getting the disease each year is slowly dropping. The WHO is aiming to put an end to TB by 2030.

Influenza

Influenza, or the flu, is a disease that is caused by a virus. It is mostly spread through the air from person to person by activities such as coughing. It can also be spread when people touch surfaces where droplets of the flu virus have landed. Flu symptoms include fever, sore throat, aches and pains, coughing and tiredness.

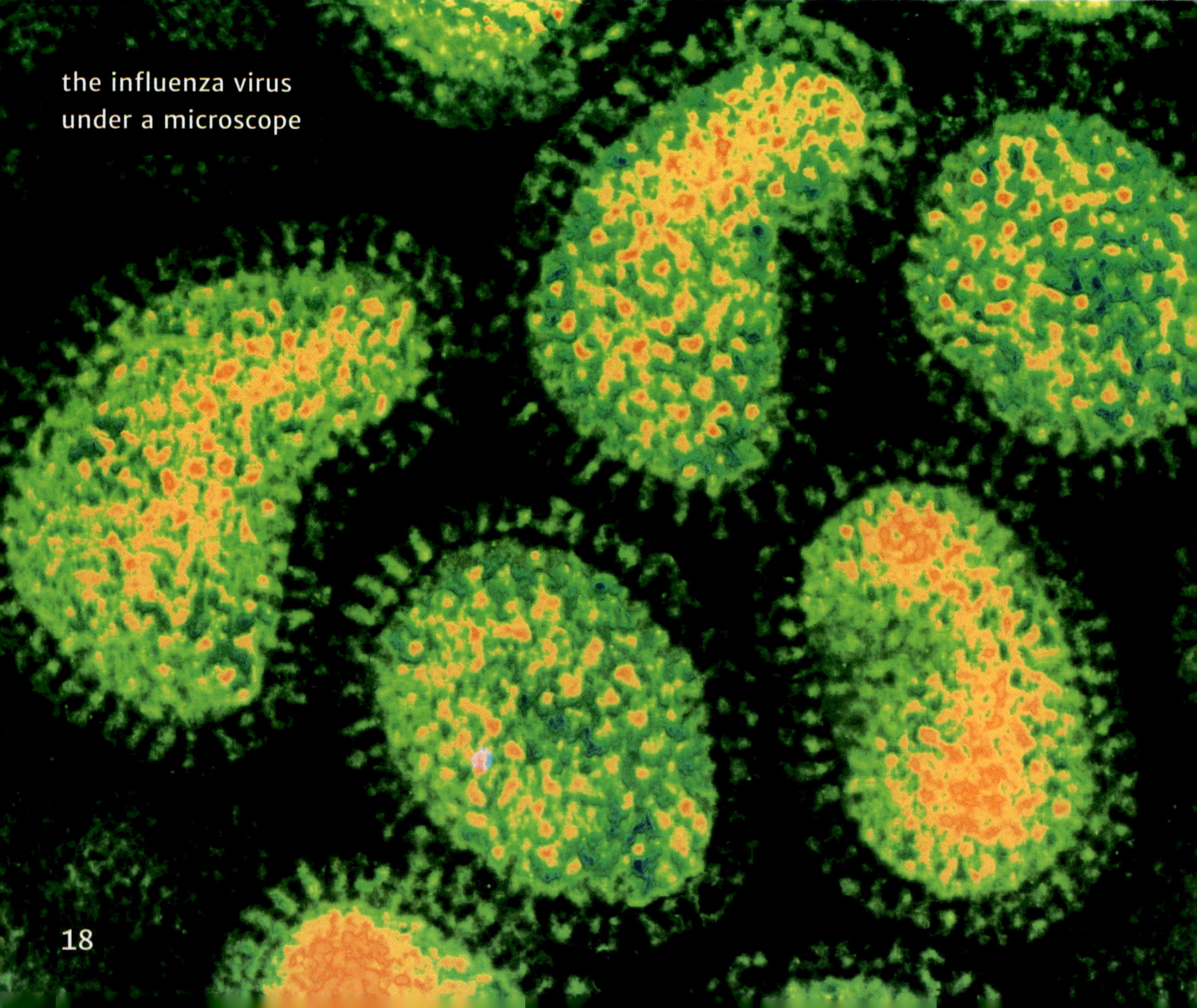

the influenza virus under a microscope

Influenza over Time

The influenza virus has existed for thousands of years. The worst known flu pandemic occurred in 1918–19 and resulted in the deaths of 25 million to 50 million people worldwide. Flu pandemics also occurred in 1957 and 1968, but they were not as deadly.

Each pandemic was caused by a new type, or "strain", of flu. Once the pandemics ended, these strains did not die off. Instead, they became milder, so fewer people were affected. While most people have protection from the flu through natural immunity and vaccination, up to 500 000 people around the world still die from the flu every year.

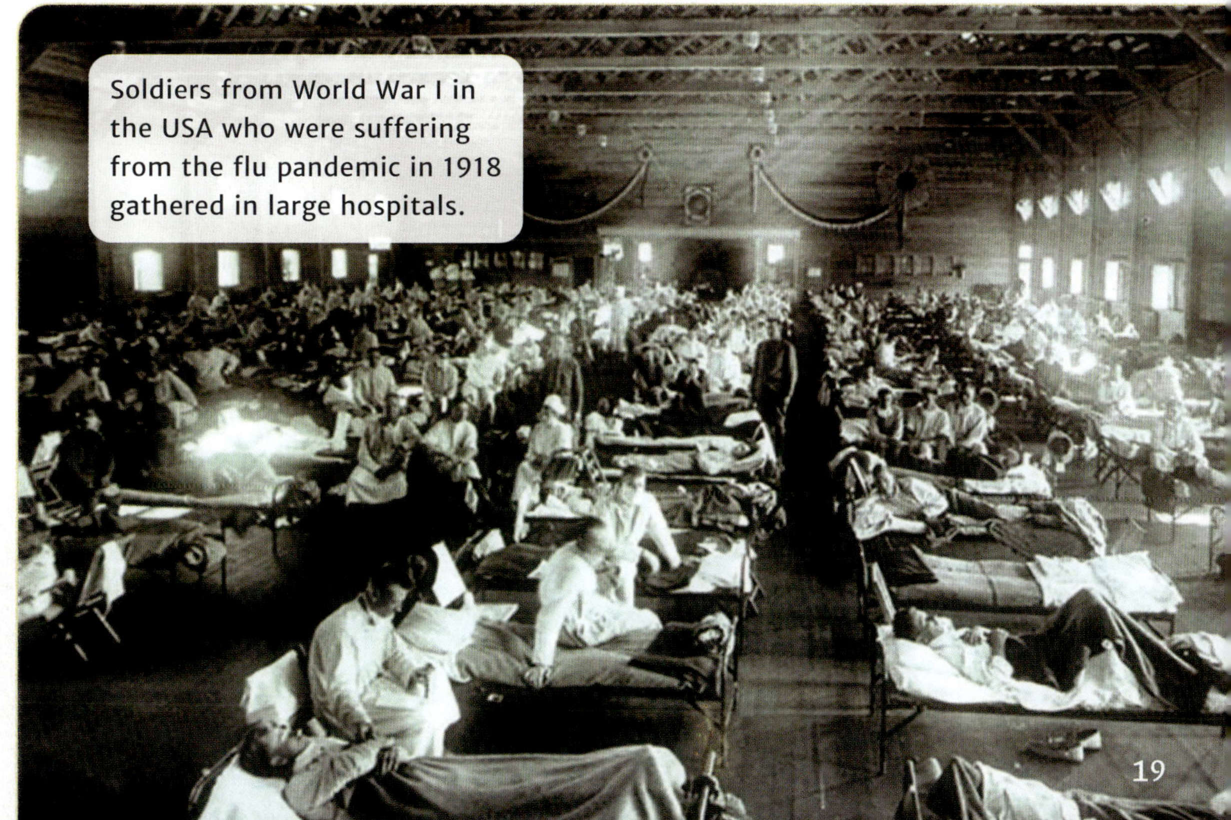

Soldiers from World War I in the USA who were suffering from the flu pandemic in 1918 gathered in large hospitals.

Thomas Francis Jr, a US research scientist, studied influenza in the 1930s. Francis helped to discover that influenza was caused by a virus, and that different strains of flu were caused by changes to the virus. He and another scientist named Jonas Salk, who went on to make the **polio** vaccine, created the first vaccines for flu in the early 1940s.

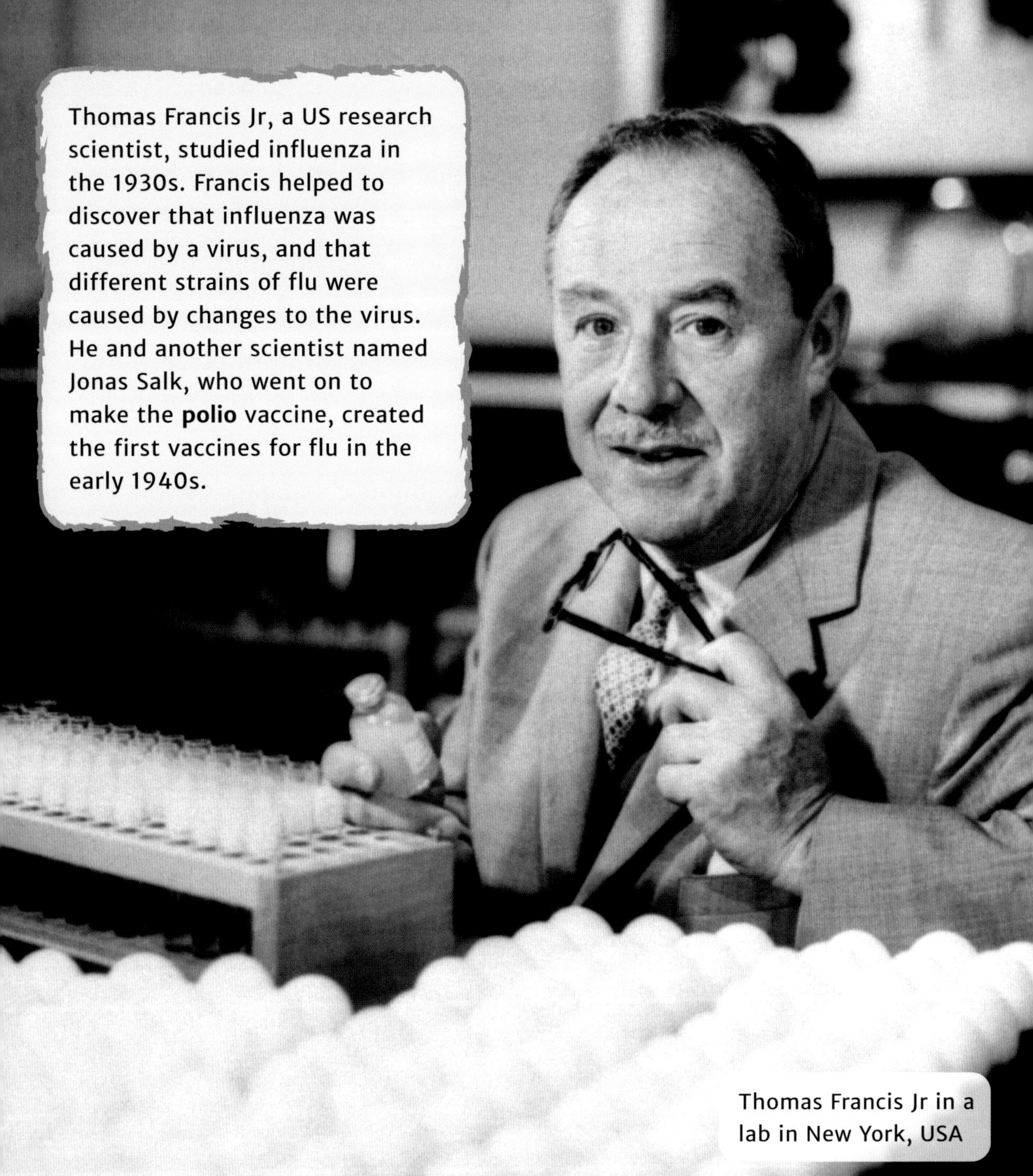

Thomas Francis Jr in a lab in New York, USA

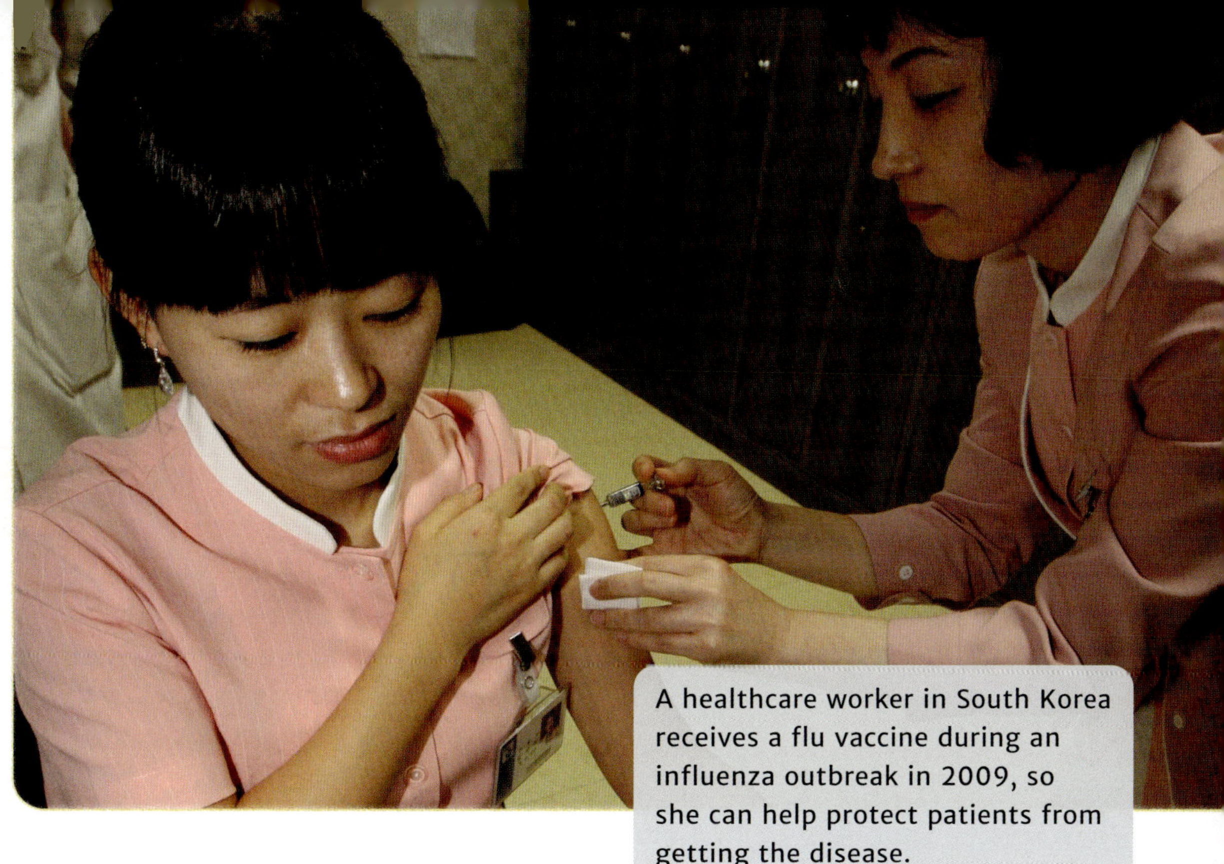

A healthcare worker in South Korea receives a flu vaccine during an influenza outbreak in 2009, so she can help protect patients from getting the disease.

Living with Influenza

Today, influenza is a seasonal illness that usually strikes in winter. Although flu vaccines do not always stop people from becoming ill, they do reduce the effects of the disease. While only about half of all adults get the flu vaccine every year, vaccination is strongly recommended for older people, those who are ill with other diseases and healthcare workers. There are also **antiviral drugs** that people can take if they become very ill with the flu, which can help with recovery. People can help prevent the flu from spreading by practising good hygiene, such as handwashing and covering their mouths when coughing and sneezing.

Malaria

Malaria is a disease caused by a tiny parasite that is passed on to people through mosquito bites. It can take up to 15 days after being bitten for people to become ill. Symptoms include chills, fever, sweats, and aches and pains. Malaria can be found in places where people live close together near **stagnant** water, which attracts mosquitoes. Malaria is a disease that can come and go in waves, and it can be present in a community for a long period of time.

Until the 1800s, it was believed malaria was caused by something nasty in the air. The word "malaria" comes from the medieval Italian words *mala aria*, meaning "bad air".

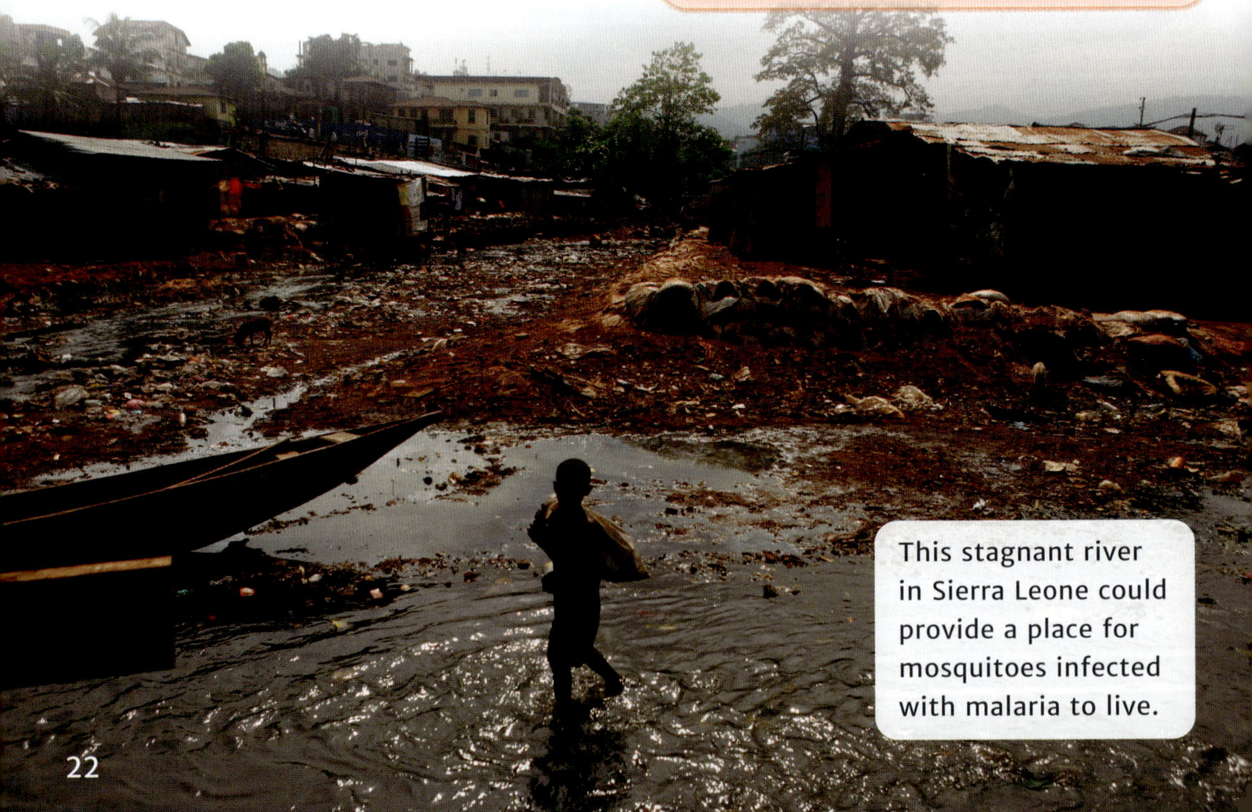

This stagnant river in Sierra Leone could provide a place for mosquitoes infected with malaria to live.

Malaria over Time

Malaria has affected humans for thousands of years and has been one of the most deadly diseases in history. In the twentieth century alone, it killed 150 million to 300 million people. In 2020, there were about 240 million cases of malaria worldwide, and 627 000 people died from the illness.

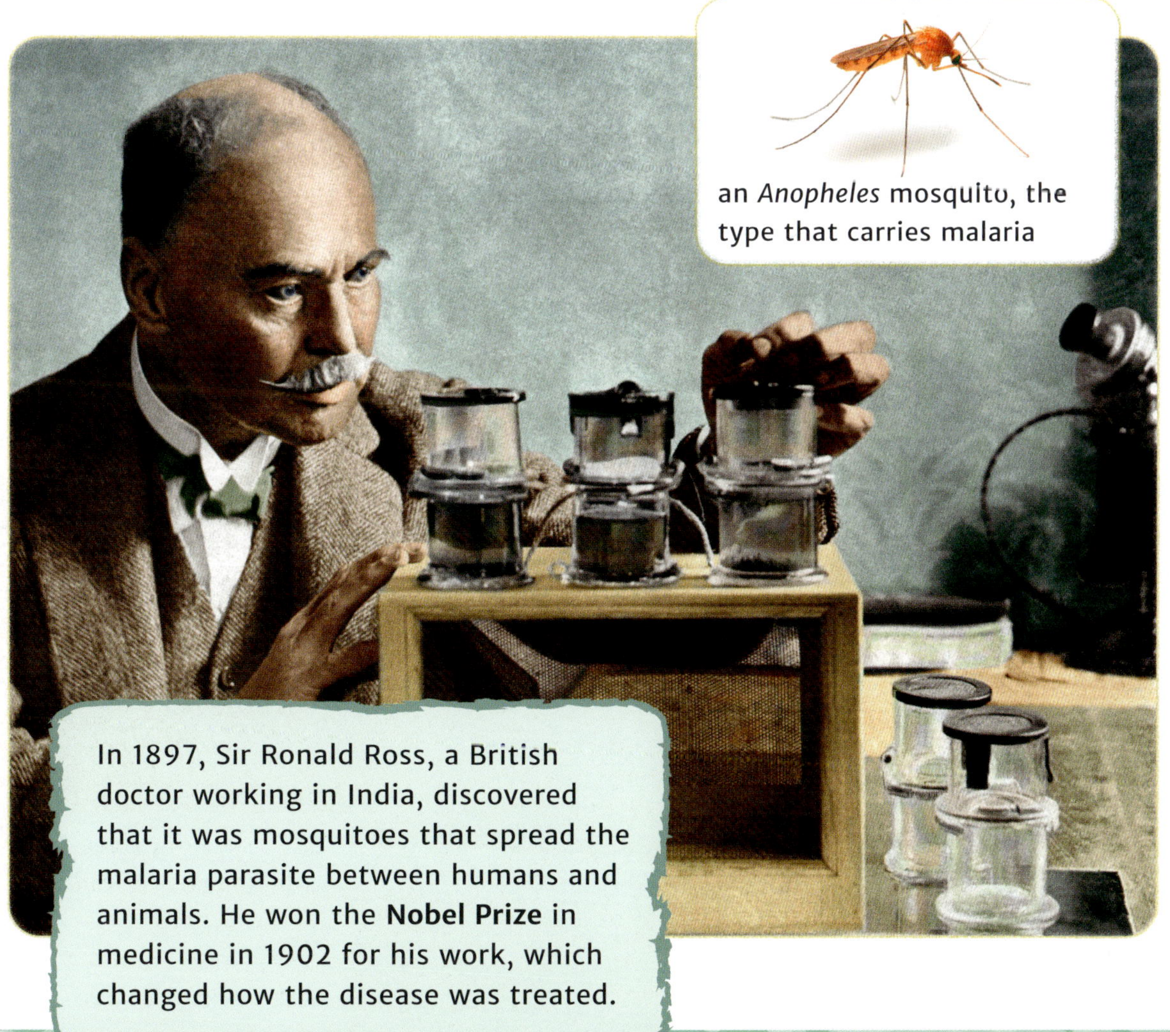

an *Anopheles* mosquito, the type that carries malaria

In 1897, Sir Ronald Ross, a British doctor working in India, discovered that it was mosquitoes that spread the malaria parasite between humans and animals. He won the **Nobel Prize** in medicine in 1902 for his work, which changed how the disease was treated.

Malaria Today

Once it was known that mosquitoes spread malaria, people were able to control the disease. This was largely done by using simple public health methods such as draining stagnant pools of water and controlling mosquitoes with nets and insect spray. A number of drug treatments were also developed to protect people from malaria and to help them recover better. In 2021, a vaccine against malaria was finally released.

However, malaria is still a problem in many countries, especially in tropical areas, where the climate is warm and wet, which makes it hard to get rid of mosquitoes. The WHO has set up the "Global Technical Strategy for Malaria" to help these countries speed up the fight against this illness. The aim is to cut cases by 90 per cent by 2030.

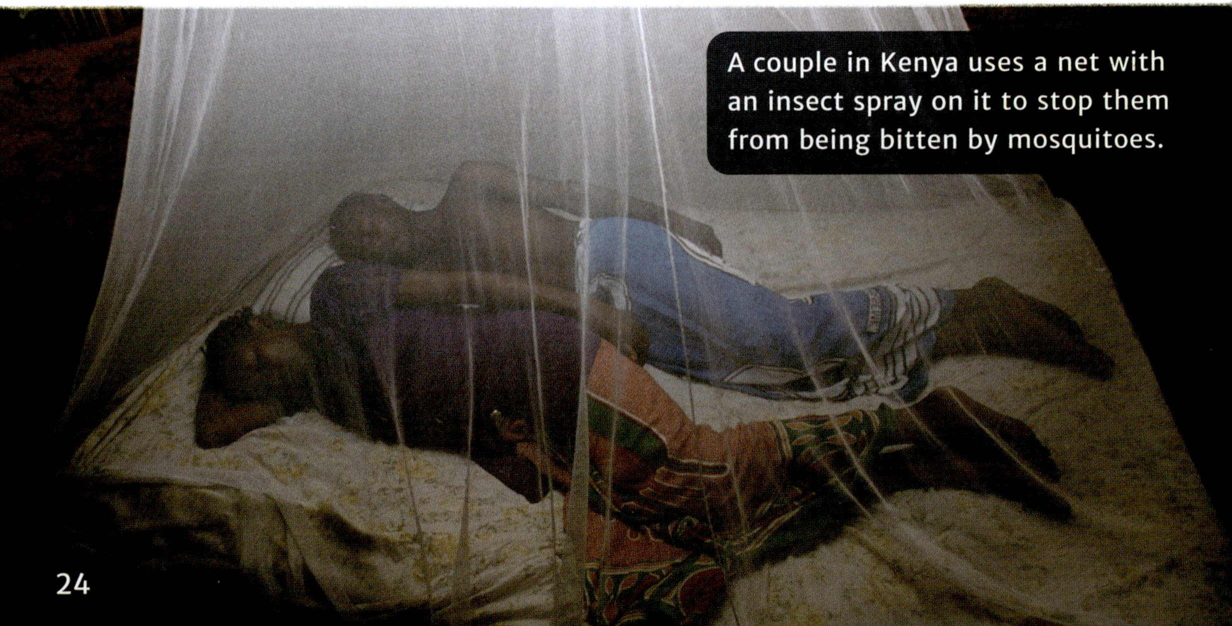

A couple in Kenya uses a net with an insect spray on it to stop them from being bitten by mosquitoes.

Covid-19

Covid-19, which is short for **co**rona**vi**rus **d**isease 20**19**, is a flu-like illness that is caused by a type of virus called a "coronavirus". Some forms of coronavirus also cause the common cold. Covid-19 is mostly passed from person to person through the air by speaking, sneezing or coughing. While some people have few or no symptoms, others can experience coughing, fever, chills, aches, headaches and loss of taste and smell. Some people can become very ill and may die.

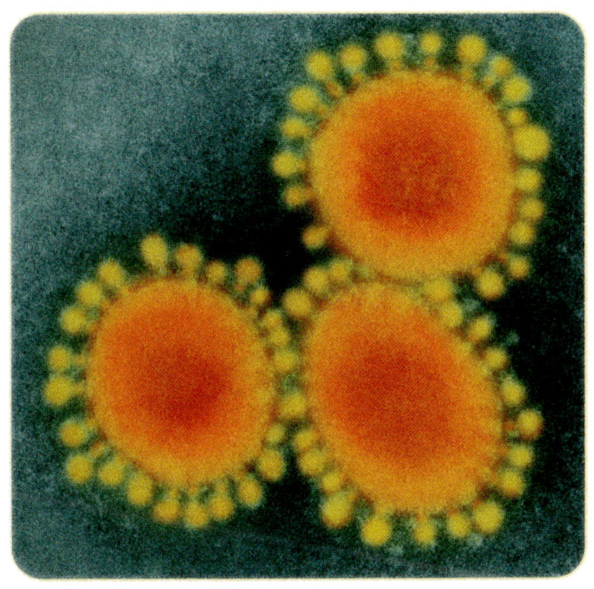

the Covid-19 virus under a microscope

Covid-19 over Time

After Covid-19 appeared in China at the end of 2019, it quickly spread to other parts of the world. Between 2020 and 2022, hundreds of millions of people caught the disease, and at least seven million people died. While most people recover quickly, some remain ill with "long Covid", which is a disease that occurs in about one in ten people who get Covid-19. The symptoms of long Covid include headaches, aches, tiredness, breathing problems and being unable to think clearly.

Covid-19 Today

Before vaccinations were released, the spread of Covid-19 was slowed down by using a range of public health methods. These included wearing masks, handwashing, physical distancing, and working and learning from home. Since then, high levels of vaccination, natural immunity and milder strains of the virus have all helped to make Covid-19 less deadly.

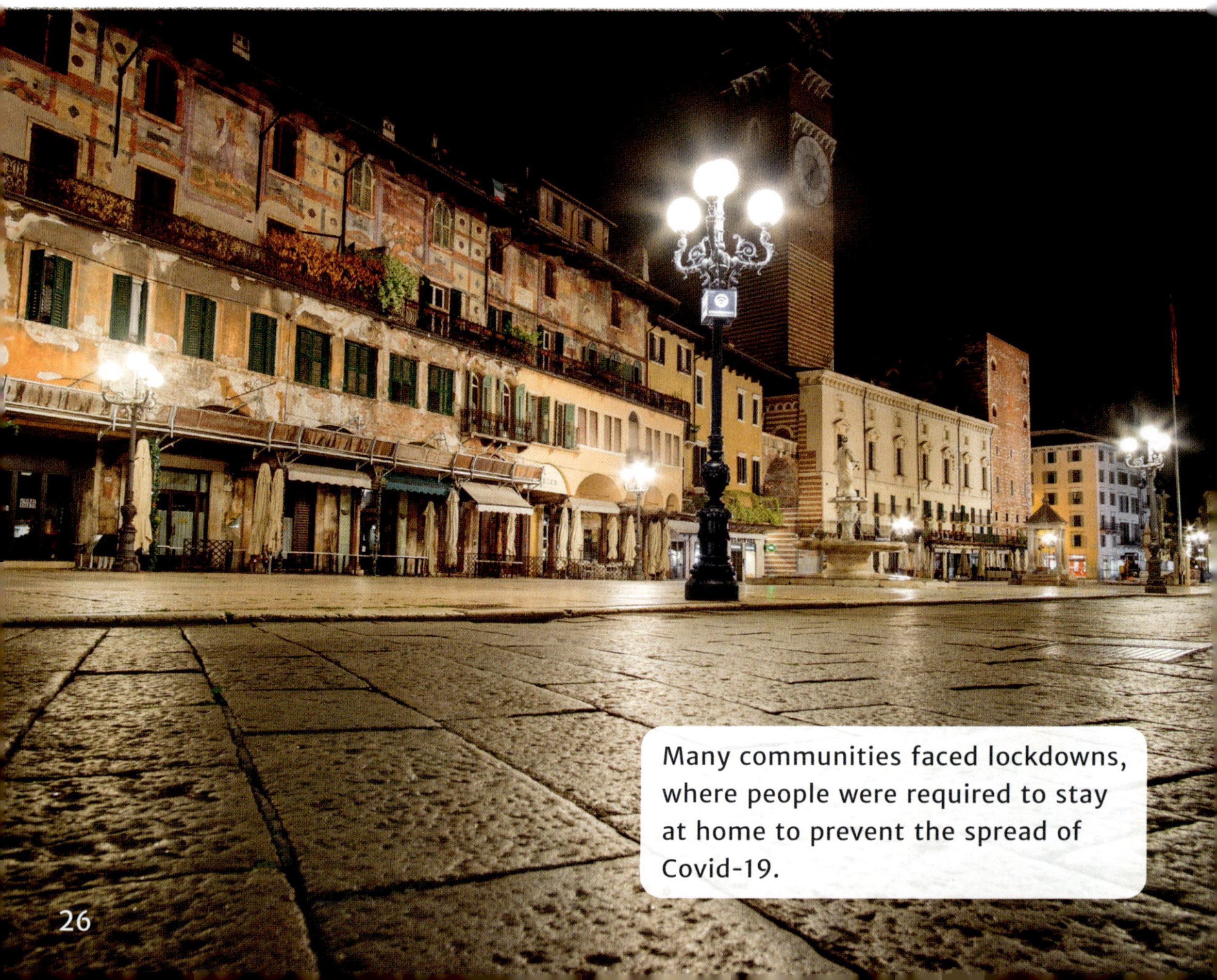

Many communities faced lockdowns, where people were required to stay at home to prevent the spread of Covid-19.

Zhang Yongzhen is a Chinese scientist who studies viruses. He identified the Covid-19 virus when it first appeared in China, and he posted information about it online for other scientists around the world to use. This helped create a number of Covid-19 tests and vaccines, which helped to make the pandemic less deadly.

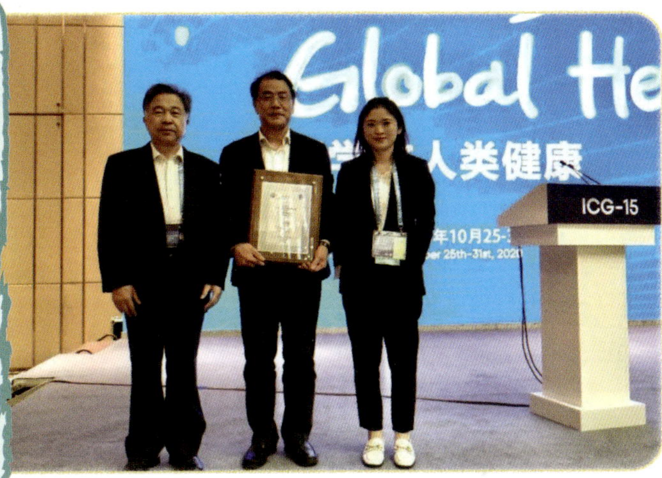

Zhang Yongzhen (middle) receiving an award for his work on the Covid-19 virus

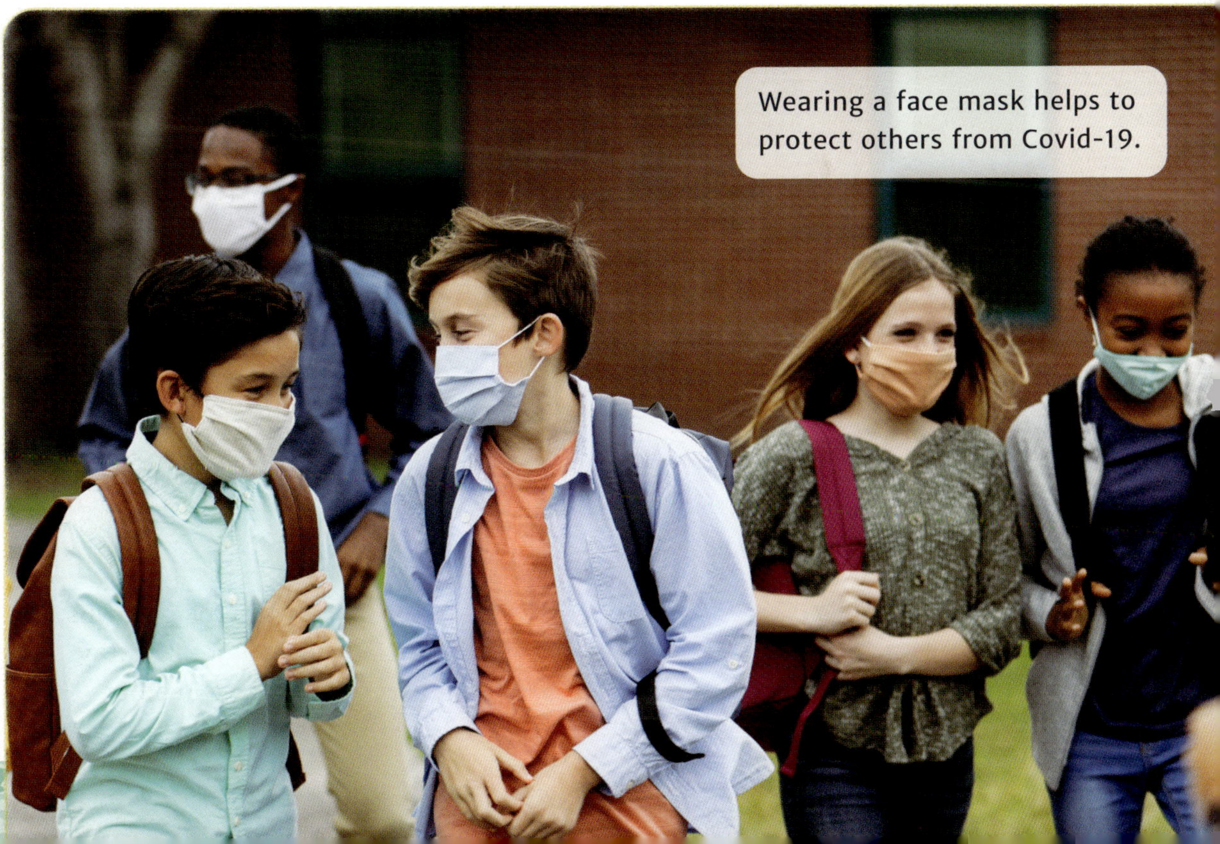

Wearing a face mask helps to protect others from Covid-19.

A Timeline of Infectious Diseases

5000 BCE: TB exists in the Mediterranean region, according to findings by modern archaeologists.

3000 BCE: Malaria exists in Egypt, according to studies of mummies from this period.

1000 BCE: Smallpox exists in Egypt, according to studies of mummies from this period.

100: Malaria is first seen in Europe, having spread from Africa and Asia.

541: The first recorded outbreak of bubonic plague begins.

1200s: Smallpox, though already in Africa and Asia, is first seen in Europe.

1347: The deadliest outbreak of bubonic plague begins.

5000 BCE | 3000 BCE | 1000 BCE | 100 CE | 1000 | 1100 | 1200 | 1300

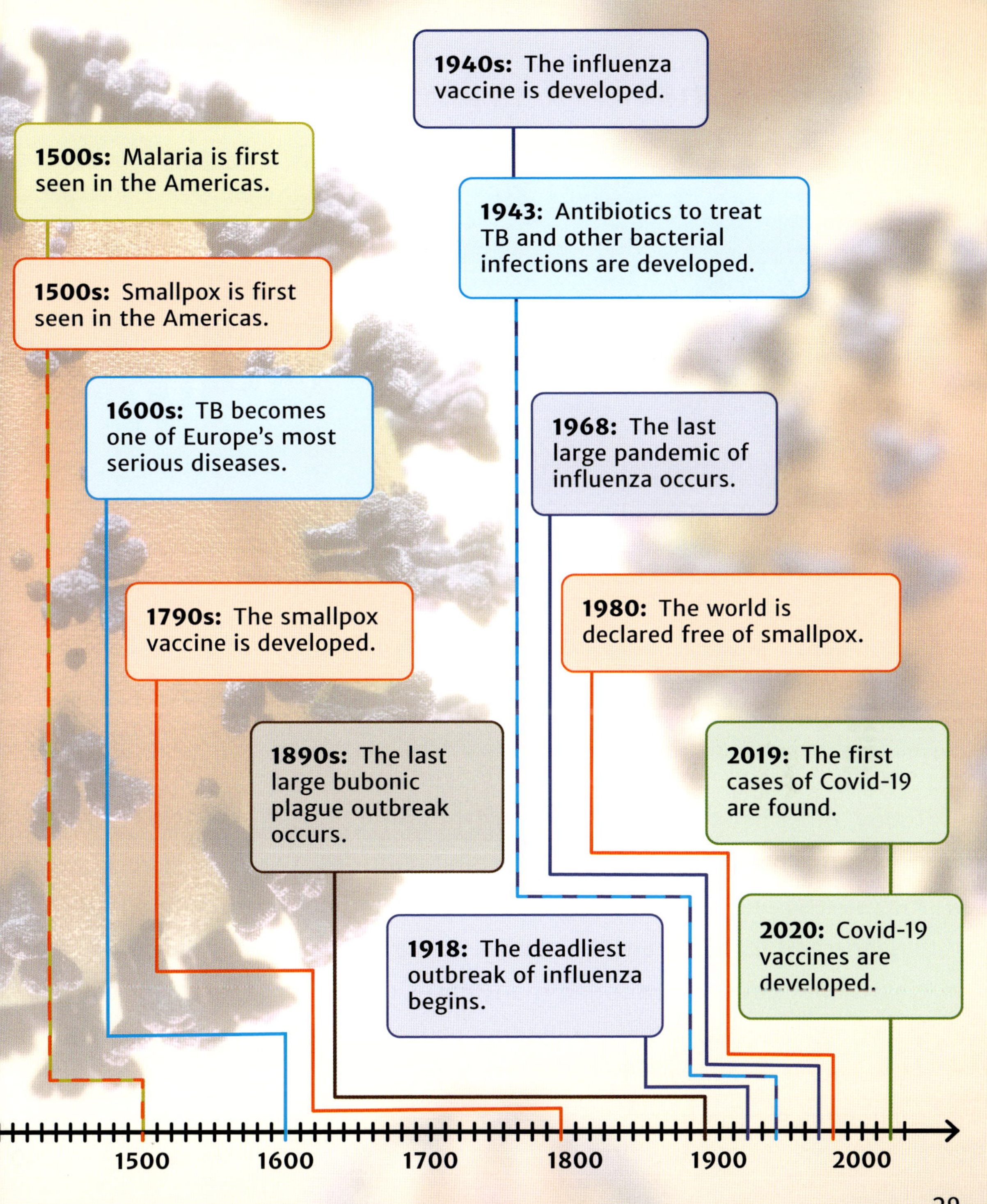

1500s: Malaria is first seen in the Americas.
1500s: Smallpox is first seen in the Americas.
1600s: TB becomes one of Europe's most serious diseases.
1790s: The smallpox vaccine is developed.
1890s: The last large bubonic plague outbreak occurs.
1918: The deadliest outbreak of influenza begins.
1940s: The influenza vaccine is developed.
1943: Antibiotics to treat TB and other bacterial infections are developed.
1968: The last large pandemic of influenza occurs.
1980: The world is declared free of smallpox.
2019: The first cases of Covid-19 are found.
2020: Covid-19 vaccines are developed.
1500
1600
1700
1800
1900
2000

Infectious Diseases Today and in the Future

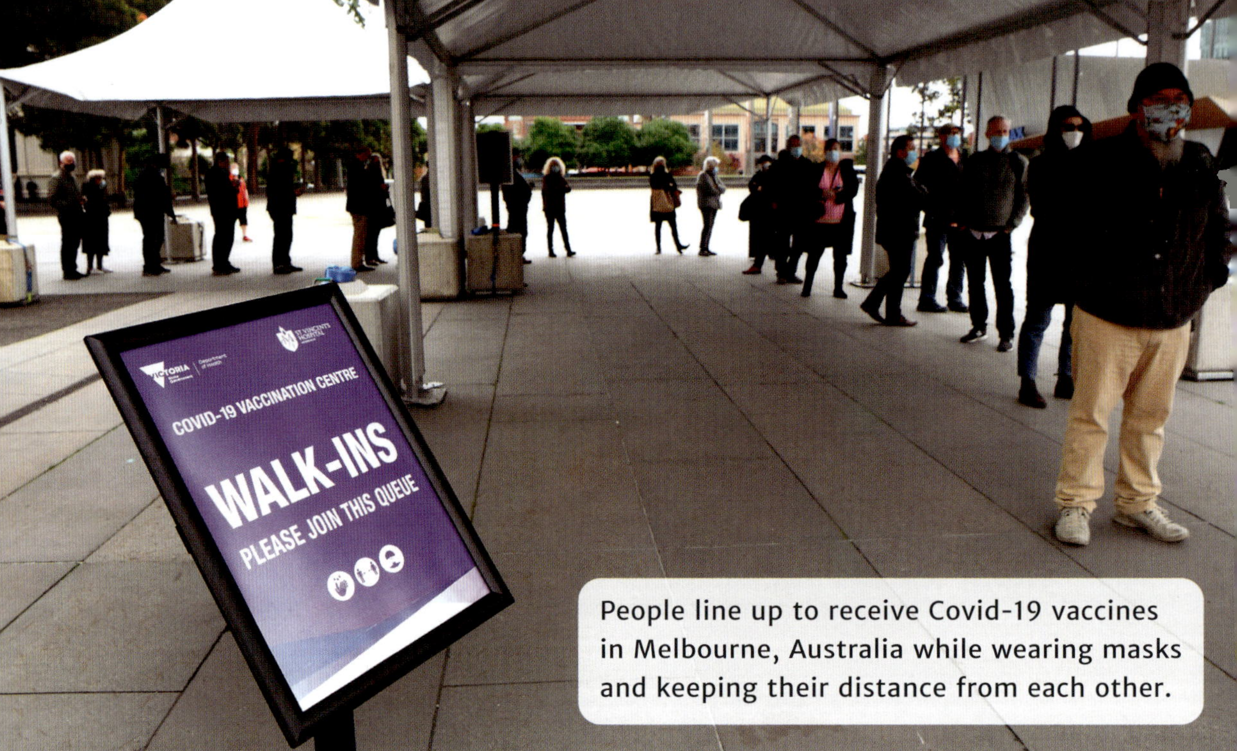

People line up to receive Covid-19 vaccines in Melbourne, Australia while wearing masks and keeping their distance from each other.

Today, most people are much safer from infectious diseases than they were a few hundred years ago. Learning about these diseases and how they spread has allowed people to control many of them with simple hygiene and public health measures. Vaccines and other medical treatments have also stopped many cases of serious illness. However, infectious diseases are still a leading cause of death in some places, and new diseases, such as Covid-19, will continue to appear, creating challenges for the future.

Glossary

antibiotics (*noun*) medicine that helps to fight illness caused by bacteria

antiviral drugs (*noun*) medicine that helps to fight a virus

bacteria (*noun*) tiny living things found in all natural environments

BCE (*adjective*) Before the Common Era; the number of years before the time dates are counted from

CE (*adjective*) years since the beginning of the Common Era

hygiene (*noun*) ways to stay clean and help prevent disease

Nobel Prize (*proper noun*) an international award for great achievements

pandemic (*noun*) when an infectious disease affects one or more countries or the whole world at one time

parasites (*noun*) living things that stay on or inside another living thing

polio (*noun*) an infectious illness causing muscle weakness

sewerage (*noun*) a way to drain waste water

stagnant (*adjective*) not flowing, or not having a current

symptoms (*noun*) signs of a disease or illness in a person

vaccines (*noun*) types of medicine to help someone build immunity to a disease

viruses (*noun*) tiny living things that can only grow by living in something else

World Health Organization (WHO) (*proper noun*) a group that helps to stop disease and promote health all over the world

Index